THE TAO OF

HEALING

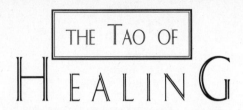

THE TAO OF
HEALING

Meditations for Body and Spirit

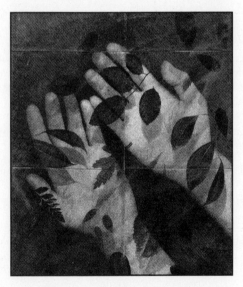

HAVEN TREVIÑO

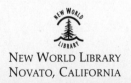

NEW WORLD LIBRARY
NOVATO, CALIFORNIA

New World Library
14 Pamaron Way
Novato, CA 94949

Revised edition © 1999 by Haven Treviño
Original edition © 1993 by Haven Treviño

Cover design: Mary Ann Casler
Typography: Tona Pearce Myers

Library of Congress Cataloging-in-Publication Data
Treviño, Haven, 1951-1993
The tao of healing : meditations for body and spirit /
Haven Treviño.
p.   cm.
Adaptation of : Tao te ching (with a focus on healing).
ISBN 1-57731-111-6 (acid-free paper)
1. Meditation-Taoism   2. Healing   I. Lao-tzu. Tao te ching.
II. Title

BL1923.T74   1993   92-44807
299'.51482-dc20   CIP

First revised printing, June 1999
Printed in Canada on acid-free paper
Distributed to the trade by Publishers Group West

10 9 8 7 6 5

For Oscar, Mona Lisa,
Siciliana, Christopher Adam, Eliza,
and all the children.
Share your gift!

FOREWORD

WHEN I first read *The Tao of Healing,* I was surprised. Instead of writing about how to heal or be healed, Haven Treviño, through his detailed adaptation of the *Tao Te Ching,* immersed me directly in the healed state.

I was reminded of what many people call "Buddha consciousness" and of the experience St. Paul describes when he writes, "Let that mind be in you which was also in Christ." Treviño seems to be saying, "Instead of practicing getting there, why not practice being there?" If nothing else, this saves us from a grating and halting process that can be antithetical to healing.

I think of this book as an invitation to dive into a string of shimmering pools. No sooner do I surface than I see before me yet another pool even more restful and lovely than the last. Disease is a process. Healing is a process. Yet this book sings of love now, wholeness now, God now. After all, God's name is I Am, not I Will Be.

I recommend that you suspend all judgment and analysis as you explore this book. Read it in stillness and comfort and with complete emptiness. Let it embrace you. Let it absorb you. Let it do the work.

There is no place to go and nothing to do. God is already here. Within the rain is the blooming. Within the thorn is the rose. And within all our stumblings are the arms of God into which we fall.

Remember that Haven Treviño was in the last stages of Lou Gehrig's disease when he wrote this book. He had already seen that only the mind can be healed. Physical changes may or may not take place as a result of mental healing, but perfection can never be found in the body. To me, his priceless gift is his insight that beneath the shell of tragedy is the pearl of God — regardless of what happens to the shell. Thus it truly can be said that Haven Treviño was a healer who healed himself. Let us take his example to heart. Let us relax into our pain. Let us relax even into our agony. And as we have been promised by so many before us, in this complete release we will begin to feel the peace that is beyond all understanding.

— Hugh Prather
author of *Spiritual Notes to Myself*

PREFACE

WHAT a special privilege and honor it is to write a few words for Haven Treviño about his very precious book, *The Tao of Healing*. This adaptation of the *Tao Te Ching* is truly miraculous in its power, depth, simplicity, and beauty. Haven came to our Center of Attitudinal Healing in Tiburon, California and was a powerful inspiration to all who knew him. He did not feel he was a victim of amyotrophic lateral sclerosis. When you were with him, you didn't see his body, you only saw and felt his heart. He truly walked his talk.

Reading this book is like listening to the heart of the universe sing an ancient melody of truth and wisdom; it is as if I am hearing a symphony of music in my ears. And it reminds me of seeing and experiencing the wonderment of Nature at its finest: I experience the stillness of the forest and the rushing of the stream, and my consciousness is uplifted beyond the wonderful and beautiful words of the printed page. It's like the feeling of awe in watching a flock of birds high in the sky flying close together, certain and clear that the direction they are traveling in is their way home.

The emphasis in this book is on healing and wholeness and the unlimited capacity that each of us has to give and receive Love. It is a book that keeps us in the present and helps us to let go of preoccupation with the past and future. Over and over again it helps us look past the body and its symptoms and focus on the compassion of the heart and the healing that takes place when we open our heart and invite Love in. It is about going inside, healing ourselves, and being of service to others.

It is about giving and receiving, Loving and forgiving, and simply being. It is not about analyzing and judging ourselves or others, but instead helps us to let our spirit soar beyond any self-imposed limits.

This is not a book to be gobbled up at one sitting. Each page is like a beautiful flower that stands erect in its own magnificence and is breathtaking to behold. Each page needs to be approached gently and slowly digested and enjoyed.

The Tao of Healing is simply one of the most beautiful books about Love that I have ever read. I only hope that you may enjoy the reading of this book as much as I have.

— Gerald G. Jampolsky, M.D.
Founder, Center for Attitudinal Healing
Tiburon, California

ACKNOWLEDGMENTS

THANKS to the wonderful staff at the Center for Attitudinal Healing in Tiburon, California, for their sensitive support and encouragement.

I would also like to thank all those who helped and blessed me along the way, especially Erin and Ronnie.

INTRODUCTION

*T*HE *Tao of Healing* is my adaptation of the *Tao Te Ching*, or "Way of Life," which first appeared around 600 B.C., and is attributed to the Chinese sage Lao Tzu. A contemporary of Confucius, Lao Tzu is thought by many to be a world teacher on the level of Christ and Buddha, and the *Tao Te Ching* has been translated more times than any other book in history, with the exception of the Bible.

I first discovered the *Tao Te Ching* in the Feng/English translation (1972). I was completely enthralled and captivated by the simple, irreducible wisdom it offered. Years later, I enjoyed reading and putting to use John Heider's *Tao of Leadership*, an adaptation of the work with a focus on business. This renewed my interest in the classic, and gave me the idea to do an adaptation with a focus on healing.

I didn't actually begin writing, however, until I went through a life-changing experience: I was diagnosed with A.L.S. — Lou Gehrig's disease — and given by doctors just a few years to live. When first diagnosed I had no idea of the journey upon which I was about to embark; it was a journey which would gradually expose the layers of fear sequestered in my rapidly deteriorating body.

As I write, I am in the "final stages" of the illness. What I have learned (and am still learning) is this: Beneath our shells of pain and darkness lives a light that transcends description, and all it takes to reunite us is our intention to do so. This light, or love, is who we truly are, and true healing is remembering this simple truth. For me, this knowledge has been the gift behind the illness, and I am grateful to be able to share some of the facets of this gift with you.

Lao Tzu spoke of the highest qualities and values to be found in the ideal leader; the highest is to be one with the Tao, or "essence of being." These same qualities apply to the healer and to the person who wishes to be healed. Each verse in this book offers a specific perspective on healing as a natural art — as the inevitable result of the intention to love.

Some thoughts on word usage: When I use the word *God,* I'm not referring to the patriarch of the Old Testament. As is clear in the text, I am referring to the essence of being, also called *Tao.* I use the term *God* because I believe that, beyond its current social and spiritual controversy, the sound carries a real vibrational meaning for our collective consciousness, similar to *I am*, *Om*, or *Amin*. More importantly, I think it is time to stop projecting our fear and rage on "God," take responsibility for our own inner separation, and finally heal this relationship. Other references to divinity I leave to your own interpretation, and capitalization of certain words such as "self" or "love" occurs usually to make an appropriate point.

Enjoy!

— Haven Treviño
January, 1993

The self is deathless.
Why?
Because life transforms into life
And Love never dies.

Before the birth of the physical
There was the birth of potential.
Before potential, something primal.
A Beingness. One Life, silent,
    unmoving, unchanging,
The unspoken beauty of Truth,
Mother only to Itself.

It has been called God, Tao,
    Divine Mother,
Universal Mind.
Today it feels good to call it Love.
Or perhaps Spirit of Love,
Since Spirit implies an all-pervading
    greatness
As common as one's breath.

Love is not an emotion, or a feeling.
It is the formlessness and substance
   permeating
The seen and the unseen;
It is the seed and womb of the
   universe.
Call it what you will, it resides
Just beyond the limits of our
   abilities to describe.

It has been said "God is Love."
Thus, the Heavens seek Love
Earth seeks Love

People seek Love.
This is what makes us great.

People abide on the Earth
Earth abides in the Heavens
The Heavens abide in Love.
Love abides in all.
This is what makes us One.

TRUE healing defined, is limited,
And so is not true healing,
As our concepts of God and Goddess
Are just that, only concepts.
Truth has no gender or division.

Before creation, Wholeness.
Healing was born of the womb of
    duality,
And whether a person is ill or well
Living in darkness or enlightenment,
It is the same.
Only our dreaming divides them.
The essence of both is ever-new joy.

Joy blossoming into joy:
The Mother and Father of all things.

3

THE pendulum swings to and fro
From darkness to light
From sickness to health
From goodness to evil
And back again.
It's enough to make anyone confused.
The sage has found the stillpoint
    between;
Remaining neutral
She teaches by living a simple,
    honest life;
She creates by allowing,
She feeds without forcing,
And gives by receiving.

She heals by perceiving
One's inner wholeness,
Then lets go.
Because she lets go,
She's always in touch.

4

THE God of this world is sometimes
   male
Sometimes female,
Lives in mountains, valleys, or heavens,
According to fashion or need.

But the God that can be conceived
Is not the One
Which holds all
Unfolds all
Fills all
Wholes all.

It is the clear light
That illuminates all colors,

The unnameable Source
Conceiving the inconceivable.

In the natural world
Sacrifice is meaningless,
As all things come and go
From the One.
The true healer,
Immune to false sacrifice,
Faces birth and death with equal joy.

All That Is, like You
Breathes in, breathes out.
The more it releases
The more it takes in.
Much talking about healing
Will stifle you.
Be still and breathe.

6

THE Breath of Life inspires
The eternal womb of the
    Divine Mother
Who conceives and gives birth
To the promise of God in every being.

Thus our well is eternal
The Breath of Life fills us
Again and again.

THE self is deathless.
Why?
Because life transforms into life
And Love never dies.

A whole person
Centered in the Self
Has no need to be self-centered.
Receiving all from the Self
Returns all,
Does not try to own life
And so becomes life.

Attune yourself to personal energy
Feel it flow like water,
Jagged stones of firm belief
Smoothed into nothing;
Cleansing, clearing, nurturing,
    healing.
Follow it faithfully, honestly,
    spontaneously,
Let it empower and serve.

Emotions are energy, too.
When they flow the most
They hurt the least.

Does a tree send its roots
   to the skies?
Will you continue to pursue
What is before your eyes?
When seeking love from another
Dare you love yourself
As much?

Life is the teacher of wisdom
So live it.
Love is the teacher of healing
So be it.

10

Truth without compassion
   is not the whole truth
And healing without a loving spirit
   is not true healing.

A miracle is merely the truth
   of God made plain
Healing is merely our separation
   from God made whole.

There is no difference between
   healer and healed,
Both must be willing to dismiss the
   ego's banal struggle

And recognize the utter holiness
Of each breath, of all things.

This is the challenge of love.

The true healer lets go of the senses
And moves from the center of intuition;
Blameless, she gives herself permission
To be exactly who she is.

PEOPLE come together to form a
    healing circle,
But the power lies in the empty center.

A person's chest rises and falls
But the breath that fills it cannot
    be seen.

Muscle and bone join to make a body
But the life force within is invisible
    to the eye.

A child's laughter bursts with joy
And the source of it cannot be
    touched.

What can one be
But the instrument of unseen bliss?

Rely on your eyes
You will not see;
Rely on your ears,
You become deaf;
Address only symptoms
And you will miss the point;
Stride after perfect health
And become lame.

The true healer lets go of the senses
And moves from the center of
    intuition;
Blameless, she gives herself
    permission
To be exactly who she is.

13

ONE who believes in success
Is no different than one who believes
  in failure:
Both have left their center.
One who heals to attain power
Is like one who suppresses symptoms;
Both are attached to the outcome.

One who identifies with a body
Will never make it whole,
But when the healer sees beyond
  the body
Healing comes naturally and without
  effort.

Know your path to be the path of all,
That you may safely guide.
Love all beings as members of your
own Body,
That you may truly serve.

You can't see it with the ordinary eye
You can't hear it with the ordinary ear
You can't feel it with the ordinary
    touch
You can't separate it from light or
    dark
You can't approach it from ahead or
    behind.

It's like a pyramid of mirrors.
Everywhere you look
You see yourself.
Open the pyramid to see what's inside:
The reflection of You.

To define your life is futile;
Don't get ahead of yourself
Don't get behind yourself
Don't compare yourself.
Just be you and enjoy what's inside.

Consider it:
In this present moment God chooses
    to be you.

15

ANCIENT Healers were one with
    infinite love
But they ignored social convention
So people thought they were crazy.
They would pay attention to what
    others overlooked;
While others debated, they would
    be silent
While others would worry, they'd
    be unconcerned.

Alert, they discover the world anew
    with each footfall
Humble, they greet you with the
    innocence of a child

Patient, they wait for nothing,
    knowing everything is here
Present, they respond to change
    like an eagle in flight
Open, they listen without judgment
Gentle, they cradle your soul in the
    memory of light.

Intent on deepest healing
Some carry the deepest wounds.
Placid, they are the still, clear pool
Reflecting mountain and sky.

16

Quiet the mind
Be still
And watch the breath of God
Rise and fall
In all things.
Allow God's breath
To be your breath;
Allow God's nature
To be your nature.

The nature of God
Is to love and be loved;
Your desire to love creates intention,
Intention focuses attention,

Attention illuminates understanding,
Understanding manifests forgiveness,
Forgiveness is the fountainhead
    of Love.

Intend to be Love
And know death for what it is:
The inbreath of God.

17

THE greatest healer
Stays in the background
Orders no one
Talks little
Loves much.

If you do not trust those you serve
How will they trust you?
Share your heart,
It's all you have
And all they need to learn.

WHEN the Way of Love is lost,
Rules and ethics are praised,
Knowledge and style worshipped
And credentials are king;

When security is sought
A professional mask appears;
For the fearful and faithless,
Associations and saviors arise.

I F all the scientists, analysts, and
    theorists disappeared today,
Not one part of truth would be lost.

If all the judges, lawyers, priests and
    prosecutors disappeared,
Not one part of morality would be lost.

If all the investors, speculators,
    and brokers disappeared,
Not one part of wealth would be lost.

On the contrary, truth, love,
    and abundance
Would be more easily received.

Center yourself first in Wholeness
And all the parts will be yours.

Live on the fine edge between
light and shadow
And infinite creation is yours.

20

APPEARING unscholarly, slovenly,
  weak,
Full of contradictions
I owe nothing to no one.

While others mask their fear
With pomp and circumstance,
Loud music and assumed poses,
I move without plan or purpose
Celebrate unseen life
With the secret smile of a child.

Perhaps I am confused,
But why own land

When the Universe is mine?
The learned declare great wisdom —
How small and foolish I feel
When I consider the cosmos.
Great minds are full
Of facts, figures, and brilliant ideas;
How worthless my contribution:
An empty slate.

Some stand out in bright display
But I am like a wave on the sea,
Who can distinguish me from all the
    rest?
Constantly,

Important people are doing important
  things.

Useless, I recline placidly
On the ample lips of the Great Mother.

21

THE Spirit of Healing, like an infinite
  cloud
Takes the moment's perfect form,
Yet is formless;
It can be seen, but not touched
Felt, but not held;
Light on the outside, dark within.

Yet even the darkness is teeming with
  life,
And failed knowledge bears the seeds
  of faith.

Therefore, allow faith to reveal;
In the last, the First is seen
In disease, Wholeness
In a blade of grass, all of creation.

22

When the Great Wheel turns
Who can stand against it?
The rigid break apart,
Therefore, relax and merge.

Yang flows into Yin and becomes
    empty;
Yin filled, becomes Yang.

Energy flows to the opposite pole,
Thus wealth flows to the simple
And the rich man's money goes out
    with the tide.

The true healer honors life.
Using the silent language of the heart
She does not speak, yet is understood,
Not promoting herself, people are
      drawn to her,
Not seeking safety, she is secure,
By serving others, is served by all,
By being ordinary, rises to perfection.

It is true:
Live on the fine edge between light
      and shadow
And infinite creation is yours.

23

THE cloud does not insist upon
    its form,
The wave does not force its way over
    the ocean,
So why should you clutch so tightly
Your little map?

Follow your heart
And know joy in all things.
The path of freedom
Has no markers,
Yet leads to fulfillment;
The path of confusion
Is crowded with signs,
Pointing in all directions.

The Great Way is a humble, solitary
    path
Leading home;
Follow it closely and be guided.
How do you know you are on the
    Way?

When your map no longer serves you.

24

TRY to stand above others
And end up on your knees.
Try to get ahead of others
And fall behind yourself.
Trying to prove yourself to others
Means you don't know who you are.
Present a facade to the world,
And you'll live to see it crumble.
Boasting of cures heals no one,
While proclaiming special powers
Will fool some and annoy others.

Spiritual arrogance is a heavy burden
     indeed;

It looks light, but is hard to bear.
Being honest is much easier
And less annoying.

No matter how great you pretend to be,
It is not as great as you truly are.

25

IF you rely on the power of another
You weaken your own.
If you seek to own the world
You limit your abundance.

The expert guide leads people forward
By plopping them on their rumps,
Dropping the contents of their minds
Down to their bellies.
Removing their goals
Strengthens their intentions.

With a clear mind
They see the confusion desire creates.

Be still and let it happen.

26

THE bird who learns to fly
Must also learn to land.
She flies far
But never forgets her nesting place.

She travels far
Yet understands her boundaries.
She appreciates external beauty
But does not compare herself to it.

The healer is like this.
She channels great joy
And avoids putting on airs;
She visits distant realms
And knows contentment's at home.

One who flits about seeking peace
Forgets to look in her own tree.

27

THE forgiving person carries
   no burdens,
Walks with a light step;
One who has no attachments
   perceives perfection
Even in the burning of her own house.

See the smoke?
Everything moves toward God.

Those who live without judgment
Have unshackled their souls
And know the unmeasured tally of
   eternal suns.

The compassionate person loves Self:
Each deed a graceful act of unthinking
  kindness.

The lover naturally sees each person as
  lovable
And in the untouchable an opportunity
  to embrace.

The fearful judge healer and wounded
  alike,
But each one wounded has the heart of
  a healer
And each healer has known a wounded
  heart.

The liberated soul sees disease
As another remarkable journey.

Fear not, friend:
There is something to be gained
From every illusion.

28

Firmness is incomplete
Without softness to receive it.
Embrace these two,
And a child is formed,
Perfect, innocent, and free.

Give to the day
Receive from the night;
Honor these two,
Become the ritual of life.

Live your highest aspirations
In an unassuming way:
Cupped hands at the crystal spring.

Be the lump of clay
And the sculptor too:
A universe of unlimited potential.

THE universe conforms
To no one's design
Nor can you heal someone
Against their will.

Their purposes are sacred,
Inviolate, encompass realms
Even illumined masters
Dare not tread.
Some are here to celebrate
Others to mourn;
Some here to be sick,
Others to be healed;
Some are here to live,

Others to die;
Some are here to love,
Others to be loved.

One who understands makes no
   attempt
To solve the puzzle of another,
To stop their world from turning
To keep a soul from learning.

30

THE healer knows
We heal no one
We cure no one;
To attempt a cure
Denies the truth:
Disharmony sown in spirit
Reaps imbalance in the flesh.

To regain the point of balance
Only open your heart,
Merely offer your life;
Allow the Love to heal,
Allow the weak to grow;
Say "I am the healer,"
You step out of the flow.

For the Universe flatters no one,
But merely offers its Life
When you offer your own.

Be centered and know eternal flow:
Not to save your life,
But to savor it.

31

Machines are not healers
When they help us forget our higher
    nature.

Fear aborts intuition,
Birthing a mechanical god.
Can machine repair spirit,
Monitor the presence of love?
Can it hold the hand of a man on the
    brink
And usher his soul into peace?

Fear of death is the only illness,
The harbinger of quackery and greed.

Those who attack plague as an enemy
    force
Wield swords of ignorance, arrows of
    despair;
Rejoice the defeat of each disease,
Wonder the coming of five more;
They applaud the saving of the body,
Oblivious to the soundless *exeunt* of
    the soul.

True healers spend little time on
    symptoms,
Rejoice only the opening of a heart.

32

THE Way of Love is infinitely large
And infinitely small.
Bring its light into your world
And watch everything
Fall smoothly into place;
The Mother and Father of All Things
Would conspire on your behalf:
A gentle rain
Of unstrained mercy and joy.

The Mother and Father of All Things
When labeled, judged, divided,
    structured,
Become prisoners

Locked in little minds.
They agree to imprisonment
They agree to enlightenment
They always say *Yes*.

It is the *Yes* of coming Home
To an open door
A warm hearth.

It is wise to yield to another,
Divine to yield to the One within.

A great thing indeed to be the ruler of
    nations,
Greater still to be the gentle master of
    your own being.
Inner peace is true abundance,
The poor in spirit seek mere authority.

Be centered and know eternal flow:
Not to save your life,
But to savor it.

Daily, without toil
Mother Earth offers her bountiful
     harvest.
Life springs from every nook and
     cranny,
Feeds and animates all
Regardless of religion or reputation.

All we have
All we are
From All That Is.
A gift.

One without wonder
Will not see It
While the eyes of the grateful
Will reflect It.

PEER behind the curtain of time
Part the thin veil of illusion
Travel to the kingdom
Beyond good and evil;
The journey of no distance.

Tempting, colorful, dramatic
The carnival of earthly play;
Drab by comparison
A discussion of the Way.

Unseen, unheard, unlimited.
A pageless book:
The story of us all.

To build up
Dismantle first
To expand
Contract first
To attain clarity
Allow confusion
To become civilized
First live in the wild.

The balance of all things
Is in their opposites;
The truth points in both directions.
Thus the clenched fist holds weakness
    within

And the open hand offers the hidden
power of suns.

Deny one-half yourself,
Stand precariously on one foot.

Love does not enter unless invited
So never meets resistance;
Creative energy flows naturally
From a state of rest;
Thus the Spirit of Love penetrates all
In its motionless embrace.
Earthly creators, reflecting this
Watch each dream come true.

Strong desire creates rigid structure,
The abode of our painful separation.
Accepting the pain of separation
Dissolves the illusion of God's
    rejection.

THE ignorant claim secret knowledge
Hoard it in a sealed chest
And suffocate.
Knowing his heart
To be his source of power
The healer shares it,
Unfolding the rose.

Outwardly, a healer does nothing.
Inwardly, a physician does nothing.
By withdrawing, the healer unifies;
Through intervention, the physician
    divides.
The less one does, the less there is to do.

The more one does, the more one
    needs to do,
And original error multiplies.

The healer offers love and
    empowers the soul.
The physician offers concern and
    treats the body.
The orderly glares at the patient and
    enforces procedure.
Thus, when love is denied
Concern is dispensed
When concern is denied
Procedures must be followed to the
    letter.

Procedures alone are a mouthful of
    chaff,
Impossible to swallow.
Prognosis comes next, attempts to
    dictate the Tao
And deny the miraculous.
What folly!

Therefore, the healer parts the shade
And reveals the light,
Sees past the pain and into the heart,
Reaches through the chaff to cradle
    the blossom.

39

LIFE is eternal and everywhere
Yet remains a quality precious,
Treasured and rare.

Receive the quality of openness and
    know clarity,
Centeredness, and know focus,
Playfulness, and know joy;
Receive the quality of humility
And know the greatness of Life.

Without openness there is separation
Without centeredness, interference
Without playfulness, decay

Without humility, the endless repetition
of pain.

Humility is the highest blessing of
Life;
Through it the great serve the lowly
And the lowly serve the great.
In this way the Universe ever uplifts
itself:
The endless nativity of Light.

RETURNING to Wholeness is the
    natural way;
Allow, allow, allow.

The choice to Love
Is the Mother of Everything.
There are no exceptions.

In silence the teachings are heard;
In stillness the world is transformed.

THOSE who know Love
Know its facility in all matters;
Others find it useful occasionally
While the broken-hearted bitterly laugh
And deny Love altogether.
Can you hear in their laughter
The sound of Heaven?

God is not to blame for the separation.
He has never turned His back on you.
Blame is the disease
Which blinds you to unity's truth.

Wake up; the nightmare is over.
The light is in them

As well as in you.
The thinnest of veils
Divides the two.
You are one Self.

You are not weak, but strong.
You are not limited, but unlimited.
You are not unloved, but much beloved.
You have suffered only for this:
That you may bless those who suffer
    still.

42

In the beginning, a Voice whispered
"I Love You . . . pass it on."

And so the seamless became sectioned
Each embracing the other
Each containing the seed of the other
And the One.

Thus we live, each seeking balance
A remembrance of Harmony
Amongst all creation.

Eons of worldly pain
The desolate march

The vale of tears
The pall of forgetfulness
Merely the Mother's bittersweet
Moment of labor:

The foreplay of unspeakable joy.

43

To penetrate the hardest armor,
Use the softest touch.
Yielding melts resistance
Density is filled by light
Good work accomplished without
    effort.

In silence the teachings are heard;
In stillness the world is transformed.

44

Would you rather be known by
    others
Or know your self?
Is making money more important
Than freedom?
Is security sought more than service?

The greedy get the least
The stingy lose the most
The fearful fare the poorest.
The one willing to give all away for free
Only grows richer.
The one who gives his life to love
Has nothing to lose.

45

"If it isn't broken, don't fix it."
The Universe isn't broken
And neither are You.
So don't attempt to fix others
Until you realize that you yourself
    are perfect.

The lame man's crutches
Are as much a part of him
As the wind
The birds
The sea.

Meditate on this
And watch the complicated grow simple.

If you're hungry, eat.
If you're tired, rest.
Stop tampering with Life
And enjoy the ride.

Will peace be found
In the sound of a dropping bomb
In the city center,
Or in the gentle plop
Of horse droppings
In a farmer's field?

Fear breeds greed
Greed, control
Control, discontent.
Disaster is the result.

Feed yourself and never have enough;
Feed others and never go hungry.

THE beauty of all existence
Rests within you:
Heaven peers from your two eyes.
Compare yourself to another,
Watch how quickly the light goes out.

Thus, when you see beauty within
You'll see it without;
As heaven shows
The healer knows.
Unconditional love has no opposite.
This is true balance.

Science constantly adds to medical
  knowledge.
It gets so complicated, who can
  understand it all?
Love is very simple,
It requires no thought or deed in order
  to work.

Anyone can do it.
Master the art of letting love happen.

Love's rule is One,
Man's rules are many.
Delusion and pain are a tangle of rules
While peace has no limitation.

49

LOVE flows into a clear mind
Ripples outward to those in need.

Your kind deeds, your loving thoughts
Travel invisible pathways,
Elevate rulers and ruled alike
A world, even worlds away.
Likewise, your faith
May light a thousand cities
Endowing both the kindly and the cruel.

Strength in one is strength in all
And light in one brings light to all.
The truth about yourself is healing.
Don't hold anything back.

50

Lose focus on life
And enter death's realm.
The body,
Full of holes
Where deadly plagues may enter;
Arms and legs,
Subject to the sword;
The erring ego held fast to the wheel
Death after death.

The illusion is this.
There is no ego,
There is only the fear the ego creates.
You cannot fear death,

For fear *is* death.
You cannot choose between
Life and death,
For there is only life.

One who walks permeated with life
Fears neither plague nor sword nor sin,
Sees death as the artifice of man.

51

WE spring forth from the All,
Fed by light,
Clothed in matter,
Sculpted by streams of inspiration,
We shape Love like the eagle shapes
    the wind.
Returning at last to the Sun,
We bring only our joy of flight.

When the Mothering Spirit
    gives birth,
Her light effortlessly feeds, shelters,
Nurtures, and uplifts.
So the true healer

Nurtures but does not control
Shelters but does not imprison
Guides others to the edge of the cliff
But does not force them to fly.

52

ONE Mother, many women.
One Father, many men.
One Spirit, many bodies.

Love the Mother in your self,
She's found in the eyes of all creation.
See Her in others,
And you'll know Her, your Self,
The triviality of death.

In life, be a listener.
Keep an even temper,
Avoid boastful displays.
Respect yourself and be tolerant of
    others.

Don't try to control or merge
With everything you see.
This brings tranquility, stability, and
    harmony.

In the small things,
See the Mother's touch.
Remember that Nature prefers
    adaptation
To domination.
Seek your inner light,
And trust it to guide you Home.

53

IT's actually much easier
And more fun
To be compassionate, kind,
Generous and forgiving.
But people seem to forget this
And wonder why they find themselves
In a world out of balance.

When we forget ourselves
We lose touch with the Earth,
Believe in powerlessness,
Invent a wrathful God
Cruel leaders
Uncaring parents

Rebellious children
A desolate world.

Your relationship with the Universe
Reflects what you remember.
There is no advantage to living in fear:
Wake up and pay attention.

A simple selfless act is a gift
Remembered by generations of
   children.

You are the source of Love.
Love your children as yourself
And live to see this light
Shine upon cities, nations, planets,
   stars.

There is no limit to what you can do.

THE healer allows Love's harmonious
   flow
Like an infant child
Soft, receiving, trusting.
But what a tenacious grip
On Mother's breast!

The babe knows nothing of sex
Yet its energy flows through the body
Shamelessly, sensitive and alive
To each pleasing moment.
Its screams and cries
Comes straight from the Source
It can cry all day and not get hoarse.

The healer is like this:
Unjudging, unafraid of Love's
    presence
Whatever form it takes.
Unflattered by power
Unhindered by shame
Unfettered by rules.

So childishly immortal:
Only the grown-up believes in death.

THOSE who know, are silent;
Those who do not, babble on forever.

Surrender your demands
Forego your dramas
Ignore magical tricks
Abandon the marketplace
Claim neither victory nor defeat;
Feel Earth living in muscle and blood.

Spoken, it loses meaning.
Lived, its power transcends limitation.

First, be kind and loving to yourself
As you would love a child;
Allow spontaneity and play in
  your work
And know the effortless healing
Of God's indiscriminate laughter.

Remember, the more complicated
  the system
The more confused the client;
The more difficult the treatment
The less likely the cure;
The more secret the method
The more scarce the love.

Remain quiet within
And they will resonate with peace;
Sow silence, and they'll reap wisdom;
Step aside, and they will heal
    themselves.

Let go your desire to heal:
Watch God emerge.

58

Love's rule is One,
Man's rules are many.
Delusion and pain are a tangle of rules
While peace has no limitation.

When fear speaks
Happiness becomes pain
And desperately people cling
To straws of sorrow.
Their left hands use magic
To repel dark spirits,
And with their fright
They invite them in again.

What is pain
But love unexpressed?
Be unshakable
But not obstinate;
Embrace fear
But do not affirm it;
Feel pain
But do not believe it.

59

WHEN channeling the forces of
heaven
The boundaries of your being create
flow,
As canyon walls transform lakes into
rivers.

The soul free from dogma
Permits an unobstructed stream:
The freer the soul, the freer the flow.

Thus, use your limits as allies
That you may produce unlimited
results;

Be open as the Mother
That the Father may enter;
To impart Heaven, be a vessel of earth.

Love like a child.
From this the rest will follow.

60

LAY on hands as you would touch a
   young child;
When the energy flows between you,
Why push hard to go deep?
When Love fills you,
Why be concerned with evil?
Dark spirits have no hold on the
   humble
And the loving healer is uplifted
By each encounter.

61

To give, receive.
Be the wet, fertile valley
That rivers of life flow through.
The full will be emptied
The empty, filled.
So be empty, that you may be filled.

The greatest healer shares all
And becomes yet greater.
One who wants to be healed
Must become a healer.
And one who wants to be a healer
Must first seek healing;

Suffering gains meaning only when
   healed
And healing is meaningless
Until it is shared.

To receive, give.

62

Words can be cheap, deeds hollow;
But when filled with truth
Reflect the glory of the One:
Irresistible pathways of focused light.

Thus when one asks to be your
        student
Don't waste your time on theory or
        style.
Teach them to respond like a master,
Love like a child.
From this the rest will follow.

Why is this way great?
Because when you ask, you receive

When you seek, you find
When you err, you're forgiven;
Endlessly and forever
No one's condemned or excluded.

Take heart!

63

IN action find stillness.
Seek the simple kernel
At the heart of every matter.
See the greatness in a small, kindly
    gesture.
Make forgiveness your intention
And your enemies are allies:
Love is perceived in all you meet.

Civilized man, afraid of Nature's
    simplicity
Creates complex problems;
The healer creates wholeness

By loving whomever God has put in
his way.

When there is trust, promises are not
required
And the difficult challenge is met
with joy.

64

HEALTH is easy to keep,
Difficult to restore;
Emotions move easily
When first they arise,
Become pain when suppressed;
To respond and release
Means less toil later.

An armored heart is easily injured
And pursuing fantasy invites despair;
A great life is composed of many
　　details,
So walk firmly — each step counts.

A grand canyon began as a tiny cleft
A great master was born a small babe;
Be happy in your place,
Growth is inevitable.
Your start and finish are the same:
The journey to enlightenment begins
Where you are right now.

One who controls
Will be out of control
And the competitive spirit
Is ever wanting.
The sage does not control
And maintains perfect balance;

She does not grab for power
So overflows with it.

The only treasure the master seeks
Is a peaceful heart;
Her only goal
To be fully where she is.
Her only doctrine
To allow.

By returning to her origins,
She brings us all forward.

65

THE World Teachers never etched
   their words
On paper or stone
For all to obey;
They knew people would only
   split hairs, bicker,
Compel others to follow their folly.

The more you listen to preachers,
The more you'll moralize and judge,
So go learn on your own.

Everything is written inside:
You are The Book.

66

Go back.
Uplift the fallen child.

There's no need to pretend anymore.
She's hurt and afraid and needs your
    help.
Set your desires aside for one moment
And see clearly what needs to be done.

You expect a child to take care of you?
Let him go and let his imagination
Teach you both.

There's no need to hide.
Declare your needs honestly

And watch the world scramble to
    assist.
Invite them in to join the celebration!

67

Some say that living in the moment
    is absurd and irresponsible.
How can you trust those who might
    harm you?
How will you survive without
    planning and toil?
How can you heal without first being
    schooled?
Fear of death,
Fear of want,
The fear of separation from God.

To choose to trust allows the fullest
    expression of life.

To choose to serve creates the greatest
   abundance.
To choose compassion brings
   Oneness and health.
Values found only moment by
   moment
Banishing all fear.
The only rational response to life.

68

THE true healer does not rush to
    judgment,
Or try to conquer disease;
He knows that simply being available
Is his greatest gift.

Not ruled by guilt,
He's not out to save the world
Or tell others how to live.

The healer opens the gates of heaven
    for others
For simple reasons:
Because he likes people
And it feels good.

69

THE precipice of vanity
Is obscured by certainty;
Tread humbly, be willing to retreat.
A confused mind is easily cleared;
Step backward, return to light.

Anger stands its ground
Insists on being right,
And the fearful maneuver
Always to save face.
Engage these and discover the
    tiresome futility
Of conversation with a mask.

View all through the clear lens of
compassion
Find the Healer behind each disguise.

70

IT is simple to feel
Yet few feel it.

It is the feeling of ancient origin
The emotion that births creation;
Available to all
Expressed by few.

The arrogant see it
Yet do not know it
And deride it,
This diamond spark that dwells
In a crude vessel of clay.

Spirit and body go hungry
When outcome takes precedence
over love.

71

SOME prefer knowing to being.
Their illness is in their heads.
Some prefer being to knowing.
Their illness is in their hearts.

She who knows her illness is
    in her heart
Is halfway home.

Denying his broken heart
No longer awed or inspired
The cynic courts disaster.
So save your high convincing talk:
He won't hear it;
In your most skilled technique
He'll find flaws.

Love all he says and all he does
Honor his arrogance and his pain
Hold him in the highest light
And fill his greatest need.

ONE man kills for peace
Another lives for it;
Yet the first man loves his dog
And beats his children,
And the other loves his children
And beats his dog.
Would you be so bold to declare
Which man Heaven loves most?

Love's flame glows
In both victor and vanquished.
Who has won?
Who has lost?
God lives in both master and slave.
Who is beating whom?

It's been written, "All that has
    happened,
Has had to happen.
All that must happen
Will happen."
So who can stand outside the circle of
    Heaven
To direct its grasp?

Look around you.
Fear of death
Is not reverence for life,
And fear of illness
Will not bring health.

Can you choose wisely
Can you see deeply
Can you touch deftly enough
To unravel this karmic knot?
Step aside and let Heaven loose,
Lest you yourself become caught
And strangle in the tangle.

Spirit and body go hungry
When outcome takes precedence
    over love.
Forget your intention to Wholeness:
Congestion in the flow.

Be willing to trust
And soar high on the mountain.
Live only for your accomplishments
And hang by the edge of the cliff
Once again.

THE young initiate is a willing
    new bud;
The jaded expert, a thicket of brittle
    thorns.
Seek new ways, and the path will
    never end;
Be certain of your knowledge
And death's around the bend.

When disease emerges
Accept, embrace, listen, respond.
Receive the blessing of those who
    suffer;

They are the heroes
Who show us the divine in ourselves.
Return the favor!

77

Wʜᴇɴ healing is the target
Illness is the bow.
What is a bow but a device for the
    transfer of energy?
Likewise an illness.

Properly used, an illness turns an
    outward focus inward,
Sends energy to where it's needed most.
Transforms fears into strength
Arrogance into humility
Compulsion to caring
Cynicism to compassion
Brings balance to imbalance.

The release of pain over-long denied.

Worldly medicine does the opposite.
It requires the patient to look
    outside herself
To give her power to another
To maintain control
To invade the body
To deny the spirit.

One who embraces illness as well
    as health
Embraces the whole of life.
She can offer life
Because she receives life.

78

WHAT is more feminine than water?
It is soft and yielding,
Yet nothing impedes
Its homeward flow to the Ocean,
And cliffs fall
Under water's constant caress.

This is obvious to all
But will you apply it to your life?

Master softness,
Don't push against the obstacle;
Yield and flow
Yield and flow.

Attack disease and invite battle;
Surrender to Love
And know true victory.

Like water, truth embraces
Both stone and starlight.

79

If someone removes symptoms,
Proclaims "You are healed!"
But imbalance remains, what good
    is that?
Better to say, "I forgive you,"
And get to the heart of the matter.
A true healer takes the challenging way,
Feeling all, accepting all, releasing all;
So becoming whole.

The Spirit of Love is impartial,
Yet only comes to those who ask.

80

A simple person leading a simple life
Knows true riches;
Living her purpose,
She's not compelled to devise a
    complicated
And gaudy life.
At peace with her many facets,
She feels no need to wander about,
Searching for what's inside.
At home with the secrets of life,
She practically ignores them
Preferring to take life as it comes.

Delighting in a kind of gesture,
A quiet moment with a friend,

She knows her sphere of influence
And fills it with light.

With the gates of heaven in her hands
She prefers to live and die right here;
For, in all the universe,
Here is where she serves.

Master. where will you seek truth,
In these flowery phrases
Or in the quiet solace of your
    own heart?
Even the ego pretends to be wise,
And whispers sage counsel in
    God's name.
Fearing death, it can never perceive
    the light.

Embrace death and receive life:
In the infinite sphere all is possible
So what is there to debate?
Living through eternity

What experience will you miss?
Having the universe at your disposal
What is there to possess?

Only the courageous surrender
    enough
To receive all the Universe has to
    offer.